# BREAST

# CANCER

# BOOK

*A Comprehensive Guide to Understanding,
Coping, Treatment, and Thriving*

*Dr. ANTHONY. WILLIAMS*

# TABLE OF CONTENTS

# 1.

# UNDERSTANDING BREAST CANCER

## Overview and Diagnosis

Breast cancer is a form of cancer that arises in the cells of the breast. It is one of the most common kinds of cancer among women globally, but it may also afflict males, although less often. Breast cancer arises when abnormal cells in the breast begin to grow uncontrolled, developing a tumor that may infiltrate neighboring tissues or spread to other regions of the body.

There are various forms of breast cancer, each with specific traits and behaviors. The most prevalent kinds are ductal carcinoma in situ (DCIS), invasive ductal carcinoma (IDC), and invasive lobular carcinoma (ILC). Additionally, breast cancer may be classed depending on the presence or lack of specific receptors, such as estrogen receptor (ER), progesterone receptor (PR), and human epidermal growth factor receptor 2 (HER2), which impact therapy choices and prognosis.

Risk factors for developing breast cancer include age, gender, family history, genetic abnormalities (such as BRCA1 and BRCA2), hormonal variables, lifestyle choices (such as alcohol intake and obesity), and exposure to radiation or specific chemicals.

Early identification via screening and timely diagnosis is critical for improving treatment results and survival rates. Various diagnostic procedures, including mammography, ultrasound, magnetic resonance imaging (MRI), and biopsy, are used to identify and confirm the existence of breast cancer, assess its stage, and guide treatment options.

**Diagnosis of Breast Cancer:**

1. **Clinical Breast Examination (CBE):** A physical examination of the breasts by a healthcare practitioner to look for any abnormalities, such as lumps or changes in breast tissue texture.

2. **Mammography:** An X-ray imaging method used to identify breast abnormalities, including tumors and microcalcifications, which may signal the existence of cancer. Mammograms are indicated as a screening technique

for early detection, especially for women aged 40 and older.

3. **Ultrasound:** Ultrasound imaging employs sound waves to provide detailed pictures of the breast tissue. It is commonly used as an additional diagnostic tool to examine abnormalities discovered on mammograms or to distinguish between fluid-filled cysts and solid tumors.

4. **Magnetic Resonance Imaging (MRI):** MRI scans give high-resolution pictures of the breast tissue and are often used in combination with mammography for women at high risk of breast cancer or to further assess worrisome findings discovered by other imaging modalities.

5. **Biopsy:** A biopsy includes the removal of a tiny tissue sample from the breast for laboratory investigation. It is the definitive approach for detecting breast cancer and defining its unique features, such as hormone receptor status and HER2 expression. Types of biopsy include core needle biopsy, small needle aspiration, and surgical biopsy.

6. **Pathology Evaluation:** Tissue samples acquired from biopsies are analyzed by pathologists to confirm the

existence of cancer, determine its grade and stage, and offer information necessary for treatment planning.

## Recent Developments in Treatment

Advances in medical science and technology have led to tremendous advances in the treatment of breast cancer. New medicines and treatment techniques continue to develop, promising greater results and quality of life for patients. Some recent advancements in breast cancer therapy include:

1. **Immunotherapy:** Immunotherapy has demonstrated encouraging outcomes in the treatment of some kinds of breast cancer, including triple-negative breast cancer (TNBC) and HER2-positive breast cancer. Immune checkpoint inhibitors, such as pembrolizumab and atezolizumab, have been authorized for use in conjunction with chemotherapy in some circumstances, harnessing the body's immune system to target and eliminate cancer cells.

2. **Targeted treatments:** Targeted treatments that selectively target molecular abnormalities in cancer cells have transformed breast cancer therapy. Drugs like trastuzumab emtansine (T-DM1) and pertuzumab have increased the therapy choices for HER2-positive breast cancer, improving outcomes and lowering the chance of recurrence.

3. **Precision Medicine:** Advances in genomics and molecular profiling have allowed the creation of tailored therapeutic regimens based on the unique genetic composition of individual cancers. Targeted medicines, such as PARP inhibitors for BRCA-mutated breast cancer, allow for more customized and successful treatment options.

4. **Minimally Invasive Surgery:** Minimally invasive surgical methods, such as laparoscopic and robotic-assisted treatments, have been increasingly employed in breast cancer surgery. These procedures provide various advantages, including fewer incisions, lower postoperative discomfort, shorter hospital stays, and speedier recovery periods compared to standard open surgery.

5. **Adjuvant treatments:** Adjuvant treatments, including hormone therapy, chemotherapy, and radiation therapy, have been developed and adjusted to decrease side effects and increase effectiveness. Advances in radiation treatment delivery, including intensity-modulated radiation therapy (IMRT) and proton therapy, allow for more accurate targeting of malignancies while preserving healthy surrounding tissues.

6. **Treatment De-Escalation and Personalized Approaches:** With greater knowledge of breast cancer subtypes and tumor biology, there is a rising focus on therapeutic de-escalation measures to limit overtreatment and eliminate needless side effects. Personalized treatment techniques try to personalize therapeutic regimens based on specific patient features, including tumor biology, genetic profile, and treatment preferences.

7. **Supportive Care and Survivorship Programs:** In addition to medical therapies, there is a growing understanding of the need for supportive care and survival programs to address the physical, emotional, and psychological needs of breast cancer patients. Integrative treatments, such as acupuncture, massage therapy, and

mindfulness-based interventions, are being increasingly introduced into comprehensive cancer care to promote general well-being and quality of life.

## Importance of Early Detection

Early identification has a critical role in the treatment and prognosis of breast cancer. Timely detection of the illness at an early stage allows for rapid action and improves treatment results. Here are a few significant reasons showing the need for early detection:

1. **Improved Treatment Options:** Detecting breast cancer early typically provides a larger choice of treatment options, including less invasive therapy such as surgery or targeted medication therapies. Early-stage breast cancers are more likely to react effectively to therapy, leading to a better likelihood of favorable outcomes and improved survival rates.

2. **Reduced Treatment Intensity:** Early identification may allow for less aggressive treatment techniques, perhaps saving patients from the side effects and consequences associated with more intensive treatments such as chemotherapy or surgery. This may

contribute to higher quality of life during and after therapy.

3. **Decreased Mortality Rates:** Studies have repeatedly demonstrated that early identification of breast cancer is related to decreased death rates. Screening mammography programs have been crucial in lowering breast cancer-related fatalities by finding cancers at an early stage when they are more curable.

4. **Smaller Tumor Size:** Breast tumors discovered at an early stage tend to be smaller in size and are less likely to have spread to surrounding lymph nodes or distant organs. Smaller tumors are often simpler to treat and may need less harsh treatment techniques.

5. **Potential for Breast Conservation:** Early-stage breast cancers may be amenable to breast-conserving operations, such as lumpectomy or partial mastectomy, saving more of the breast tissue and retaining a more natural breast look compared to mastectomy.

6. **Improved Prognosis:** Early identification of breast cancer is linked with a more favorable prognosis since the illness is less likely to have

progressed to an incurable stage. Early-stage breast cancers have a better possibility of being cured, leading to long-term survival and enhanced quality of life for patients.

7. **Empowerment and Control:** Regular breast cancer screening empowers people to take care of their health and allows early diagnosis of any anomalies. This proactive strategy allows for prompt medical intervention, providing patients with a feeling of control over their health results.

8. **Opportunity for Risk Reduction Strategies:** Identifying people at high risk for breast cancer by screening may trigger the adoption of risk reduction treatments, such as lifestyle adjustments, chemoprevention, or preventive surgery, to minimize the chance of acquiring the illness.

# 2.

# MEDICAL TREATMENT OPTIONS

## Surgery, Chemotherapy, and Radiation Therapy

Medical treatment options for breast cancer often comprise a mix of medicines suited to the particular features of the illness, including the kind and stage of the cancer, as well as the patient's overall health and preferences. Among the principal treatment options are surgery, chemotherapy, and radiation therapy.

**1. Surgery:**

Surgery is frequently the primary therapy for localized breast cancer and seeks to remove the tumor and surrounding damaged tissue. There are various surgical options for breast cancer:

- **Lumpectomy (Breast-Conserving Surgery):** This surgery comprises the excision of the tumor and a narrow margin of surrounding healthy tissue while conserving the remainder of the breast. A lumpectomy is frequently followed by radiation treatment to lower the chance of cancer recurrence.

- **Mastectomy:** Mastectomy entails the surgical removal of the whole breast. Depending on the extent of the disease and individual factors, different types of mastectomy may be performed, including total mastectomy (removal of the entire breast tissue), modified radical mastectomy (removal of breast tissue and nearby lymph nodes), or skin-sparing mastectomy (preservation of breast skin for breast reconstruction).

- **Sentinel Lymph Node Biopsy:** During surgery, sentinel lymph nodes (the initial lymph nodes to which cancer cells are most likely to spread) may be removed and evaluated to identify whether cancer has spread beyond the breast. This helps guide additional treatment selections.

**2. Chemotherapy:**

Chemotherapy is the use of chemicals to destroy cancer cells or prevent them from growing and dividing. It is frequently provided systemically either intravenous infusion or oral medicine and may be prescribed before or after surgery, depending on the stage and severity of the malignancy. Chemotherapy may also be used to decrease tumors before surgery (neoadjuvant chemotherapy) or to eradicate leftover cancer cells after surgery (adjuvant chemotherapy).

Chemotherapy regimens vary depending on individual circumstances, including the kind of breast cancer, tumor size, hormone receptor status, and general health. Common chemotherapy medications used in the treatment of breast cancer include anthracyclines (e.g., doxorubicin), taxanes (e.g., paclitaxel), and platinum-based compounds (e.g., carboplatin).

**3. Radiation Therapy:**

Radiation treatment employs high-energy beams to target and kill cancer cells. It is generally given externally by a machine called a linear accelerator and is widely used after lumpectomy or mastectomy to lower the chance of cancer recurrence in the breast or chest wall.

The major aims of radiation therapy in breast cancer treatment include:

- **Adjuvant Radiation:** Adjuvant radiation treatment is delivered following breast-conserving surgery (lumpectomy) to eliminate any leftover cancer cells in the breast tissue and lower the probability of local recurrence.

- **Post-Mastectomy Radiation:** Post-mastectomy radiation treatment may be advised for persons with specific high-risk factors, such as big tumors, involvement of many lymph nodes, or positive surgical margins, to lower the chance of recurrence in the chest wall or regional lymph nodes.

- **Partial Breast Irradiation:** In rare circumstances, partial breast irradiation treatments, such as brachytherapy or accelerated partial breast irradiation (APBI), may be employed to deliver radiation selectively to the tumor bed while sparing surrounding healthy tissues.

These medical treatment options, including surgery, chemotherapy, and radiation therapy, are commonly used in combination or sequentially as part of a complete treatment strategy for breast cancer. The selection and sequencing of therapy rely on several criteria, including the stage, subtype, and specific features of the cancer, as well as patient preferences and general health state. Close communication between patients and healthcare professionals is vital in making informed treatment choices and maximizing results in breast cancer care.

## - Hormonal Therapies and Targeted Treatments

In addition to surgery, chemotherapy, and radiation therapy, hormone therapies and targeted treatments play essential roles in the management of breast cancer. These therapy techniques are widely utilized in hormone receptor-positive (HR+) breast cancers and HER2-positive breast cancers, respectively, targeting particular molecular properties of the tumor to suppress its development and proliferation.

**1. Hormonal Therapies:**

Hormonal treatments, also known as endocrine therapies, are utilized largely in hormone receptor-positive breast tumors, where the tumor cells express estrogen receptors (ER) and/or progesterone receptors (PR). These medicines function by interfering with the hormone signaling pathways that encourage cancer cell proliferation. Common hormonal therapy for breast cancer include:

- **Selective Estrogen Receptor Modulators (SERMs):** Drugs such as tamoxifen and toremifene block estrogen receptors in breast tissue, hence decreasing estrogen-driven tumor development. Tamoxifen is routinely used in both premenopausal and postmenopausal women with HR+ breast cancer.

- **Aromatase Inhibitors (AIs):** AIs, including anastrozole, letrozole, and exemestane, lower estrogen levels in postmenopausal women by inhibiting the enzyme aromatase, which transforms androgens into estrogen. AIs are primarily utilized as adjuvant or first-line treatment in postmenopausal women with HR+ breast cancer.

- **Selective Estrogen Receptor Degraders (SERDs):** Drugs such as fulvestrant bind to estrogen receptors and stimulate their degradation, resulting to diminished estrogen receptor signaling. Fulvestrant is licensed for the treatment of HR+ metastatic breast cancer in postmenopausal women.

- **Luteinizing Hormone-Releasing Hormone (LHRH) Agonists:** LHRH agonists, such as goserelin and leuprolide, decrease ovarian function and diminish estrogen levels in premenopausal women, typically used in conjunction with other hormonal treatments or chemotherapy.

Hormonal medications are usually well-tolerated and are linked with less systemic adverse effects compared to chemotherapy. However, they may have unique adverse effects connected to hormonal changes, including as hot flashes, vaginal dryness, and bone density loss.

**2. Targeted Treatments:**

Targeted therapies are aimed to selectively target molecular abnormalities or processes implicated in cancer development and progression, enabling a more precise and individualized approach to therapy. Two primary targeted therapy are employed in breast cancer:

- **HER2-Targeted medicines:** Human epidermal growth factor receptor 2 (HER2)-targeted medicines are utilized in HER2-positive breast tumors, where the tumor cells overexpress the HER2 protein. These therapies include:

- **Monoclonal Antibodies:** Drugs such as trastuzumab (Herceptin), pertuzumab (Perjeta), and trastuzumab emtansine (T-DM1, Kadcyla) bind to HER2 receptors on cancer cells, disrupting their signaling pathways and promoting immune-mediated death of the tumor cells.

- **Tyrosine Kinase Inhibitors (TKIs):** Drugs like lapatinib and neratinib decrease the activity of HER2 tyrosine kinase, affecting downstream signaling cascades and decreasing tumor development.

HER2-targeted treatments are typically utilized in conjunction with chemotherapy or as part of adjuvant or neoadjuvant treatment regimens in HER2-positive breast cancer.

- **CDK4/6 Inhibitors:** Cyclin-dependent kinase 4/6 (CDK4/6) inhibitors, including palbociclib, ribociclib, and abemaciclib, are used in conjunction with hormone treatments to stop cell cycle progression and reduce the proliferation of HR+ breast cancer cells. These medications have showed benefit in both advanced and early-stage breast cancer, increasing progression-free survival and overall survival results.

Targeted treatments provide the possibility for more successful and less toxic therapies compared to standard chemotherapy, especially in cancers with specific molecular abnormalities. However, they may be accompanied with specific side effects related to their modes of action, necessitating careful monitoring and control.

In summary, hormonal therapy and targeted treatments constitute major pillars of breast cancer treatment, notably in hormone receptor-positive and HER2-positive breast cancers, respectively. These treatments, frequently used in conjunction with other modalities, contribute to better outcomes and quality of life for patients impacted by breast cancer.

# 3.

# EMOTIONAL AND PSYCHOLOGICAL IMPACT

A breast cancer diagnosis can have profound effects on an individual's mental health and their relationships with others. Coping with the emotional and psychological aspects of the disease is an essential part of the journey through diagnosis, treatment, and survivorship. Here's how breast cancer can impact mental health and relationships:

## Mental Health and Relationships

**1. Mental Health Challenges:**

- **Anxiety and Fear:** A breast cancer diagnosis often triggers feelings of anxiety and fear about the future, including concerns about treatment, prognosis, and how life may change. Coping with uncertainty and managing anxiety can be challenging but important for overall well-being.

- **Depression:** It's not uncommon for individuals with breast cancer to experience depression, characterized by persistent feelings of sadness, hopelessness, and loss of interest in activities. Coping with the physical and emotional toll of cancer treatment can contribute to depressive symptoms.

- **Stress and Coping:** Dealing with the demands of breast cancer treatment, such as surgery, chemotherapy, and radiation therapy, can be highly stressful. Finding effective coping strategies, such as relaxation techniques, exercise, or talking to a therapist, can help manage stress levels.

- **Body Image and Self-esteem:** Breast cancer treatments, including surgery and chemotherapy, can impact physical appearance and self-image. Coping with changes to the body, such as hair loss or mastectomy, may affect self-esteem and body image. Support and counseling can be helpful in adjusting to these changes.

**2. Relationship Dynamics:**

- **Partner Relationships:** Breast cancer can affect intimate partner relationships, with changes in communication, roles, and intimacy.

Partners may experience feelings of uncertainty, fear, and stress alongside the person diagnosed. Open communication and mutual support are key to navigating these challenges together.

- **Family Dynamics:** Breast cancer can also impact relationships with family members, including children, parents, and siblings. Family members may struggle with their own emotions and roles as caregivers or supporters. Open communication and support within the family can help maintain relationships during difficult times.

- **Friendships and Social Support:** Friendships and social support networks play a crucial role in coping with breast cancer. Some friendships may change or evolve in response to the diagnosis, while others may become stronger. Seeking support from friends and participating in support groups can provide emotional comfort and understanding.

- **Caregiver Stress:** Family members or friends who serve as caregivers for someone with breast cancer may experience stress and burnout. Caregiver stress can impact their own mental health and well-being. It's important for caregivers to prioritize self-care and seek support when needed.

**3. Coping Strategies and Support Services:**

- **Seeking Professional Help:** If feelings of anxiety, depression, or distress become overwhelming, it may be helpful to seek support from a mental health professional. Therapy, counseling, or support groups can provide a safe space to express emotions, learn coping skills, and receive guidance.

- **Mindfulness and Self-care:** Practices such as mindfulness meditation, yoga, and relaxation techniques can help reduce stress and promote emotional well-being. Engaging in activities that bring joy and relaxation can also be beneficial for mental health.

- **Open Communication:** Open and honest communication with loved ones about feelings, concerns, and needs can strengthen relationships and foster understanding. Sharing the cancer experience with trusted individuals can provide emotional support and connection.

- **Educational Resources:** Learning about breast cancer, treatment options, and coping strategies can empower individuals and their loved ones to make informed decisions and advocate for their needs. Educational resources, books, and online support communities can provide valuable information and support.

In conclusion, addressing the mental health and relationship challenges associated with breast cancer is essential for overall well-being and quality of life. By acknowledging emotions, seeking support, and utilizing coping strategies, individuals and their loved ones can navigate the journey of breast cancer with resilience and strength.

## Coping Strategies and Emotional Support

Receiving a breast cancer diagnosis can be overwhelming, bringing about a range of emotions and challenges. Coping with the emotional and psychological impact of breast cancer requires a multifaceted approach that incorporates coping strategies and emotional support. Here are some effective coping strategies and sources of emotional support for individuals facing breast cancer:

- **Therapy and Counseling:** Individual therapy with a psychologist, psychiatrist, or counselor specialized in oncology can provide a safe space to explore emotions, fears, and concerns related to breast cancer. Therapy can help individuals develop coping strategies, improve emotional resilience, and enhance overall well-being.

- **Support Groups:** Joining a breast cancer support group, whether in-person or online, offers the opportunity to connect with others who understand the challenges of the disease firsthand. Support groups provide emotional support, practical advice, and a sense of community, helping individuals feel less isolated and more empowered.

**2. Utilizing Mind-Body Practices:**

- **Mindfulness Meditation:** Practicing mindfulness meditation can help individuals manage stress, reduce anxiety, and enhance emotional well-being. Mindfulness techniques, such as deep breathing exercises and guided imagery, promote relaxation, present-moment awareness, and acceptance of difficult emotions.

- **Yoga and Exercise:** Engaging in gentle yoga, tai chi, or other forms of exercise can benefit both physical and emotional health during breast cancer treatment and recovery. Exercise releases endorphins, improves mood, reduces stress, and enhances overall quality of life.

**3. Maintaining Social Connections:**

- **Family and Friends:** Spending time with supportive family members and friends provides emotional comfort, companionship, and encouragement during difficult times. Open communication and meaningful connections with loved ones help individuals feel understood, valued, and less alone in their cancer journey.

- **Peer Support:** Connecting with other individuals who have experienced breast cancer can offer valuable insights, empathy, and encouragement. Peer support networks, survivorship programs, and online communities provide opportunities to share experiences, exchange information, and receive mutual support.

**4. Engaging in Creative Expression:**

- **Art Therapy:** Engaging in creative activities, such as painting, drawing, writing, or crafting, can serve as a form of self-expression and emotional release. Art therapy provides a therapeutic outlet for processing emotions, reducing stress, and promoting healing.

- **Journaling:** Keeping a journal or writing down thoughts and feelings can help individuals process their emotions, gain insight, and track their cancer journey. Journaling offers a private and reflective space to express fears, hopes, gratitude, and personal growth.

**5. Practicing Self-care:**

- **Self-compassion:** Practicing self-compassion involves treating oneself with kindness, understanding, and self-acceptance during challenging times. Being gentle with oneself, practicing self-care rituals, and cultivating self-compassionate thoughts can promote emotional resilience and well-being.

- **Setting Boundaries:** Setting boundaries and prioritizing self-care is essential for managing stress and preserving emotional health during breast cancer treatment. Learning to say no, delegating tasks, and prioritizing activities that bring joy and fulfillment help prevent burnout and maintain balance.

Coping with breast cancer requires a holistic approach that addresses emotional, psychological, and social needs. By seeking professional support, utilizing mind-body practices, maintaining social connections, engaging in creative expression, and practicing self-care, individuals can navigate the challenges of breast cancer with resilience, strength, and hope.

# 4.

## HOLISTIC THERAPEUTIC APPROACHES

**Yoga, Meditation, and Nutrition**

In addition to conventional medical treatments, holistic therapeutic approaches can play a valuable role in supporting individuals throughout their breast cancer journey. Practices such as yoga, meditation, and nutrition offer benefits for physical, emotional, and psychological well-being, enhancing overall quality of life. Here's how these holistic approaches can complement traditional cancer care:

**1. Yoga:**

- **Physical Benefits:** Yoga involves gentle stretching, strengthening, and relaxation techniques that can help improve flexibility, balance, and range of motion. For individuals undergoing breast cancer treatment, yoga may alleviate treatment-related side effects such as fatigue, muscle tension, and lymphedema.

- **Emotional Support:** Practicing yoga promotes stress reduction, relaxation, and emotional well-being. Mindful breathing techniques and meditation incorporated into yoga sessions can help individuals manage anxiety, depression, and emotional distress associated with a breast cancer diagnosis.

- **Community and Support:** Participating in yoga classes or support groups specifically tailored for individuals affected by breast cancer offers a sense of community, connection, and understanding. Sharing experiences and support with others in a supportive environment can be empowering and comforting.

**2. Meditation:**

- **Stress Reduction:** Meditation techniques, such as mindfulness meditation, guided imagery, and loving-kindness meditation, promote relaxation and reduce stress levels. Regular meditation practice can help individuals cultivate a sense of calm, resilience, and emotional balance amidst the challenges of breast cancer.

- **Emotional Resilience:** Meditation fosters emotional resilience and coping skills, enabling individuals to navigate difficult emotions, fears, and uncertainties related to their cancer diagnosis and treatment. By cultivating present-moment awareness and acceptance, meditation promotes psychological well-being and inner peace.

- **Mind-Body Connection:** Meditation encourages a deeper connection between the mind and body, facilitating self-awareness, self-compassion, and healing. By tuning into bodily sensations, thoughts, and emotions without judgment, individuals can develop greater insight and self-understanding throughout their cancer journey.

**3. Nutrition:**

- **Optimal Nutrition:** Maintaining a balanced and nutritious diet is essential for supporting overall health and well-being during breast cancer treatment and recovery. Eating a variety of fruits, vegetables, whole grains, lean proteins, and healthy fats provides essential nutrients, antioxidants, and phytochemicals that support immune function and cellular repair.

- **Managing Side Effects:** Nutrition plays a crucial role in managing treatment-related side effects, such as nausea, fatigue, and appetite changes. Dietary modifications, such as consuming small, frequent meals, staying hydrated, and avoiding certain foods that exacerbate symptoms, can help alleviate discomfort and promote tolerance to treatment.

- **Supporting Healing and Recovery:** Proper nutrition supports the body's healing and recovery processes, helping individuals maintain energy levels, strength, and vitality throughout their cancer journey. Nutrient-dense foods provide essential nutrients that support tissue repair, immune function, and overall health.

Incorporating holistic therapeutic approaches such as yoga, meditation, and nutrition into a comprehensive cancer care plan can enhance physical, emotional, and psychological well-being for individuals affected by breast cancer. These practices offer tools and resources for coping with the challenges of diagnosis, treatment, and survivorship, empowering individuals to thrive holistically throughout their cancer journey.

# Incorporating Holistic Practices into Daily Life

In the face of a breast cancer diagnosis, integrating holistic therapeutic approaches into daily life can offer valuable support for physical, emotional, and psychological well-being. These practices empower individuals to take an active role in their healing journey and enhance their overall quality of life. Here are some strategies for incorporating holistic practices into daily life:

**1. Mindful Awareness:**

- **Start the Day Mindfully:** Begin each day with a few moments of mindful awareness. Set aside time in the morning to center yourself through deep breathing exercises, meditation, or gentle stretching. Allow yourself to connect with your body, emotions, and intentions for the day ahead.

- **Practice Mindful Eating:** Approach meals with mindfulness by paying attention to the sensations of hunger, fullness, and taste. Savor each bite, chew slowly, and appreciate the nourishment provided by your food. Choose nutrient-rich foods that support your health and vitality.

**2. Movement and Exercise:**

- **Choose Activities You Enjoy:** Engage in physical activities that bring you joy and relaxation. Whether it's walking, yoga, dancing, or swimming, find movements that feel good for your body and uplift your spirit. Regular exercise can boost energy levels, reduce stress, and improve overall well-being.

- **Incorporate Movement Throughout the Day:** Look for opportunities to incorporate movement into your daily routine. Take short walks during breaks, stretch at your desk, or practice gentle yoga poses throughout the day to release tension and promote circulation.

**3. Emotional Well-being:**

- **Express Gratitude:** Cultivate a sense of gratitude by reflecting on the blessings in your life. Keep a gratitude journal and write down three things you're grateful for each day. Focusing on the positive aspects of your life can shift your perspective and promote emotional resilience.

- **Connect with Nature:** Spend time outdoors and connect with the natural world. Take walks in nature, sit in a garden, or simply observe the beauty of the sky, trees, and flowers. Nature has a calming effect on the mind and can provide a sense of peace and renewal.

***4. Stress Reduction:***

- **Practice Stress Management Techniques:** Incorporate stress reduction techniques into your daily routine to promote relaxation and emotional well-being. Deep breathing exercises, progressive muscle relaxation, and guided imagery can help calm the mind and body during times of stress.

- **Set Boundaries:** Learn to prioritize your needs and set boundaries to protect your physical and emotional well-being. Say no to activities or commitments that drain your energy and schedule time for rest, relaxation, and self-care.

**5. Nourishing Relationships:**
- **Cultivate Supportive Relationships:** Surround yourself with friends, family members, and support networks who uplift and encourage you. Share your thoughts, feelings, and concerns with trusted individuals who offer understanding, empathy, and validation.

- **Express Love and Affection:** Take time to nurture your relationships and express love and affection to those you care about. Connect with loved ones through meaningful conversations, acts of kindness, and quality time together.

Incorporating holistic practices into daily life is about fostering a sense of balance, connection, and well-being in all aspects of your being. By embracing mindfulness, movement, emotional well-being, stress reduction, and nourishing relationships, individuals affected by breast cancer can cultivate resilience, strength, and healing throughout their journey.

# 5.

# LIFESTYLE DURING AND AFTER TREATMENT

## Diet, Exercise, and Stress Management

Maintaining a healthy lifestyle during and after breast cancer treatment is essential for overall well-being and recovery. Adopting healthy habits related to diet, exercise, and stress management can support physical strength, emotional resilience, and quality of life. Here's how to focus on each aspect:

**1. Diet:**

- **Emphasize Nutrient-Rich Foods:** Prioritize a diet rich in fruits, vegetables, whole grains, lean proteins, and healthy fats. These foods provide essential nutrients, antioxidants, and phytochemicals that support immune function, cellular repair, and overall health.

- **Stay Hydrated:** Drink plenty of water throughout the day to stay hydrated and support bodily functions.

Limit consumption of sugary beverages and opt for water, herbal teas, or infused water with fresh fruits and herbs.

- **Manage Side Effects:** Some breast cancer treatments may cause side effects such as nausea, changes in appetite, or digestive issues. Work with a registered dietitian to develop a personalized nutrition plan that addresses these side effects and ensures adequate nourishment.

- **Limit Alcohol and Processed Foods:** Limit alcohol intake and reduce consumption of processed foods, sugary snacks, and high-fat foods. These choices may contribute to inflammation, weight gain, and other health concerns.

**2. Exercise:**

- **Incorporate Regular Physical Activity:** Aim for at least 150 minutes of moderate-intensity aerobic exercise or 75 minutes of vigorous-intensity aerobic exercise each week, as recommended by health guidelines. Activities such as walking, swimming, cycling, or yoga can improve cardiovascular health, muscle strength, and overall fitness.

- **Start Slowly and Progress Gradually:** If you're new to exercise or have been inactive during treatment, start with gentle activities and gradually increase intensity and duration over time. Listen to your body and honor its needs, pacing yourself as needed.

- **Include Strength Training:** Incorporate strength training exercises into your routine to build and maintain muscle mass, bone density, and physical strength. Use resistance bands, free weights, or bodyweight exercises to target major muscle groups and improve overall function.

- **Stay Active Throughout the Day:** Look for opportunities to stay active throughout the day, such as taking short walks, stretching breaks, or doing household chores. Every bit of movement adds up and contributes to overall health and well-being.

**3. Stress Management:**

- **Practice Relaxation Techniques:** Incorporate relaxation techniques into your daily routine to reduce stress and promote emotional well-being. Techniques such as deep breathing, meditation, mindfulness, or progressive muscle relaxation can help calm the mind and body.

- **Engage in Enjoyable Activities:** Make time for activities that bring joy, relaxation, and fulfillment. Whether it's reading, gardening, listening to music, or spending time with loved ones, engaging in pleasurable activities helps alleviate stress and promote a sense of happiness and contentment.

- **Seek Support:** Reach out for support from friends, family members, support groups, or mental health professionals as needed. Sharing your thoughts, feelings, and concerns with others can provide validation, empathy, and comfort during challenging times.

- **Set Boundaries:** Learn to prioritize your needs and set boundaries to protect your physical and emotional well-being. Say no to activities or commitments that drain your energy and schedule time for rest, relaxation, and self-care.

By incorporating healthy habits related to diet, exercise, and stress management into your daily routine during and after breast cancer treatment, you can support your body's healing process, enhance your overall well-being, and promote long-term health and vitality.

# Importance of Sleep Hygiene

Sleep hygiene plays a crucial role in maintaining overall health and well-being, particularly during and after breast cancer treatment. Adequate and restorative sleep is essential for physical recovery, emotional resilience, and quality of life. Here's why prioritizing sleep hygiene is important during and after breast cancer treatment:

**1. Physical Recovery:**

- **Supports Immune Function:** Quality sleep is essential for optimal immune function. During sleep, the body repairs and regenerates tissues, produces immune cells, and fights off infections. Adequate sleep supports the body's ability to recover from cancer treatments and maintain overall health.

- **Promotes Healing:** Sleep is a critical time for cellular repair and regeneration. Getting enough restorative sleep allows the body to repair damaged tissues, reduce inflammation, and promote healing after surgery, chemotherapy, radiation therapy, or other cancer treatments.

- **Regulates Mood:** Sleep plays a key role in regulating mood and emotional well-being. Chronic sleep deprivation can lead to irritability, mood swings, anxiety, and depression, which can exacerbate the emotional challenges associated with a breast cancer diagnosis and treatment.

- **Reduces Stress:** Quality sleep helps reduce stress levels and promotes emotional resilience. Adequate rest allows the body and mind to relax, recharge, and better cope with the stressors of cancer treatment, recovery, and life changes.

**3. Cognitive Function:**

- **Enhances Cognitive Functioning:** Sleep is essential for cognitive function, memory consolidation, and mental clarity. Getting enough restful sleep improves concentration, problem-solving skills, and decision-making abilities, which are important for managing treatment decisions and daily tasks.

- **Reduces Cognitive Impairment:** Sleep deprivation can impair cognitive function and lead to difficulties with memory, attention, and concentration. Prioritizing sleep hygiene reduces the risk of cognitive impairment and supports overall brain health during and after breast cancer treatment.

**4. Tips for Improving Sleep Hygiene:**

- **Establish a Consistent Sleep Schedule:** Go to bed and wake up at the same time every day, even on weekends. Consistency helps regulate the body's internal clock and improves sleep quality.

- **Create a Relaxing Bedtime Routine:** Develop a relaxing bedtime routine to signal to your body that it's time to wind down. Activities such as reading, taking a warm bath, practicing relaxation techniques, or listening to soothing music can help prepare you for sleep.

- **Create a Comfortable Sleep Environment:** Make your bedroom conducive to sleep by keeping it dark, quiet, and cool. Invest in a comfortable mattress, pillows, and bedding to support restful sleep. Minimize noise and distractions that may disrupt sleep.

- **Limit Screen Time Before Bed:** Reduce exposure to electronic devices, such as smartphones, computers, and TVs, before bedtime. The blue light emitted by screens can interfere with the production of melatonin, a hormone that regulates sleep-wake cycles.

- **Limit Stimulants and Alcohol:** Avoid consuming caffeine, nicotine, and alcohol close to bedtime, as they can disrupt sleep patterns and affect sleep quality.

- **Stay Active During the Day:** Engage in regular physical activity during the day, but avoid vigorous exercise close to bedtime. Physical activity promotes restful sleep and helps regulate the sleep-wake cycle.

Prioritizing sleep hygiene during and after breast cancer treatment is essential for supporting physical recovery, emotional well-being, and cognitive function. By incorporating healthy sleep habits into your daily routine, you can optimize sleep quality, enhance overall health, and improve your quality of life during the cancer journey and beyond. If you experience persistent sleep disturbances or insomnia, consult with your healthcare provider for personalized recommendations and support.

# 6.

# INSPIRATIONAL SURVIVOR STORIES

## Triumphs and Resilience Against Breast Cancer

Inspiring Survivor Stories: Triumphs and Resilience Against Breast Cancer, Presented by Breast Cancer Survivors

Breast cancer is a difficult path, but despite the challenges, innumerable stories of victory and tenacity inspire hope and courage. These experiences can be found in their entirety. Individuals who have fought breast cancer with grace and courage are highlighted in these survivor stories, which demonstrate their strength, tenacity, and perseverance. The following are some stories of survivors that are motivational:

1. Anne's Struggle from a Strength Perspective:

At an early age, Anne was given a diagnosis of breast cancer, and she is currently engaged in a challenge-filled fight against the disease. With unyielding perseverance and a positive attitude, Anne tackled her diagnosis, despite the anxiety and uncertainty that she was experiencing. Anne remained resilient throughout the entirety of her treatment journey, which included surgery, chemotherapy, and radiation therapy. She drew strength from the support of her loved ones and the community of breast cancer patients.

Anne was able to find the strength to endure each obstacle, and she refused to allow the disease to define who she was. Her attitude toward life was one of fresh appreciation; she cherished every moment and discovered happiness in the simplest of joys. Anne's resilience and optimism inspired people around her, serving as a light of hope for others experiencing similar problems.

Today, Anne is a vibrant survivor, living life to the fullest and pushing for breast cancer awareness and support. Her path is a testament to the power of tenacity, positivism, and the human spirit in overcoming adversity.

**2. Sarah's Journey of Faith:**

Sarah's breast cancer diagnosis came as a painful blow, demanding her faith and testing her resilience. As a mother, wife, and ardent believer, Sarah depended on her faith as a source of strength and solace during her cancer battle. She sought peace in prayer, leaning on her spiritual convictions to manage the uncertainties and challenges ahead.

Despite the physical and mental toll of therapy, Sarah stayed steady in her determination, trusting in a higher force and finding serenity amidst the storm. She embraced each day with thankfulness and focused on the blessings in her life and the affection of her family.

Through the darkest stages of her cancer experience, Sarah's strong faith sustained her, bringing her toward healing and optimism. Today, she is a living witness to the power of faith, resilience, and the indomitable human spirit in triumphing over adversity.

**3. David's Journey of Support:**

David's wife, Rachel, was diagnosed with breast cancer, sending their family into a maelstrom of anxiety and uncertainty. As Rachel endured treatment, David stood by her side as a pillar of strength and support, offering unfailing love, encouragement, and friendship.

Despite the hurdles they experienced, David and Rachel addressed her cancer journey as a team, drawing closer together and finding strength in their friendship. David's continuous support and dedication were important in Rachel's healing journey, providing her with the strength and comfort she needed to persist.

Through the ups and downs of Rachel's treatment, David remained a source of comfort and optimism, assuring her that she was not alone in her struggle. Together, they negotiated the difficulties of breast cancer with courage, resilience, and an unbreakable spirit of love.

These amazing survivor stories serve as reminders of the perseverance, fortitude, and courage that lay inside each fighting breast cancer. Through the power of hope, determination, and support, survivors prevail over adversity, inspiring others to embrace life with courage, grace, and appreciation.

# 7.

## SUPPORT AND RESOURCES

## Accessing Emotional Support Networks

Emotional support is a critical element of coping with a breast cancer diagnosis. Accessing emotional support networks can provide patients with a sense of camaraderie, empathy, and empowerment as they negotiate the challenges of their cancer journey. Here's how breast cancer patients can contact emotional support networks:

**1. Hospital and Cancer Center Programs:**

- **Support Groups:** Many hospitals and medical centers provide support groups exclusively for breast cancer sufferers. These groups provide a safe and supportive place for individuals to share their experiences, anxieties, and feelings with others who understand. Patients should speak with their healthcare team about available support groups and how to join.

- **Individual Counseling:** Counseling services may be accessible through hospitals or cancer centers, providing patients with one-on-one assistance from licensed therapists or counselors. Individual therapy sessions can help patients process their feelings, establish coping mechanisms, and negotiate the psychological challenges of their diagnosis and treatment.

**2. Nonprofit Organizations:**

- **Breast Cancer Support Organizations:** Numerous charitable organizations specialize in offering support services for breast cancer patients. These organizations may offer helplines, online forums, support groups, and educational resources to assist patients to connect with others, obtain information, and find emotional support. Examples include Susan G. Komen, Breastcancer.org, and the American Cancer Society.

**3. Online Support Communities:**

- **Social Media Groups:** Social media platforms feature a variety of breast cancer support groups and communities where sufferers can interact with others suffering similar circumstances. Facebook groups, Reddit forums, and

Instagram communities provide platforms for patients to share their stories, ask questions, and offer support and encouragement to one another.

- **Online Forums and Chatrooms:** Dedicated breast cancer forums and chatrooms give sufferers areas to interact with friends, share advice, and seek emotional support. Websites such as Cancer Survivors Network and Breast Cancer Now offer online forums where patients can engage in discussions and find sympathy with others on similar experiences.

**4. Peer Support Programs:**

- **Mentorship Programs:** Some organizations offer peer support or mentorship programs that match newly diagnosed patients with breast cancer survivors who have finished treatment. These programs provide patients with emotional support, practical assistance, and guidance from someone who has firsthand experience with the problems of breast cancer.

**5. Local Community Resources:**

- **Community Centers:** Local community centers may organize support groups, workshops, or educational programs for breast cancer patients and survivors. These events give opportunity for individuals to interact with others in their community, share information, and find emotional support close to home.

Accessing emotional support networks is a vital aspect of coping with the emotional burden of breast cancer. By connecting with individuals who understand their experiences and problems, patients can find solace, affirmation, and strength as they navigate their cancer journey. Whether through in-person groups, online communities, or peer support programs, emotional support networks offer vital tools and connections to help patients feel supported and empowered during their treatment and recovery.

## Professional Counseling and Guidance

Dealing with a breast cancer diagnosis can be emotionally stressful, and expert counseling and advice can provide important support to patients as they negotiate the obstacles of their journey. Here's how expert counseling and guidance might benefit breast cancer patients:

- **Processing Emotions:** Professional counselors and therapists provide a secure and non-judgmental space for patients to share their thoughts, worries, and concerns connected to their diagnosis and treatment. Counseling sessions allow patients to explore and express complicated emotions such as worry, sadness, anger, and loss, helping them cope more effectively with their cancer experience.

- **Coping Strategies:** Counselors work with patients to build personalized coping methods and approaches to manage stress, anxiety, and other emotional issues associated with breast cancer. These strategies may include relaxation exercises, mindfulness techniques, cognitive-behavioral approaches, and problem-solving abilities to increase emotional resilience and well-being.

**2. Decision-Making Support:**

- **Navigating Treatment Options:** Facing decisions about treatment options can be difficult for breast cancer patients. Professional counselors can help patients understand their treatment choices, balance the benefits and risks, and make informed decisions that line with their beliefs, preferences, and aspirations.

- **Supportive Decision-Making:** Counselors provide support and advice to patients as they navigate treatment options, delivering a sympathetic and understanding presence throughout the decision-making process. They encourage patients to advocate for themselves, ask questions, and seek explanations from their healthcare team.

**3. Relationship Support:**

- **Communication Skills:** Breast cancer can impair relationships with family members, partners, and friends. Counselors assist patients to improve communication skills and negotiate tough talks with loved ones about their diagnosis, treatment, and emotional needs. They facilitate open and honest discussion, developing understanding, empathy, and support within partnerships.

- **Couples Counseling:** For patients in love relationships, couples counseling can help partners navigate the obstacles of breast cancer together. Counselors provide a friendly atmosphere for couples to address relationship difficulties, cope with changes in intimacy and responsibilities, and strengthen their bond as they navigate the cancer journey as a team.

**4. Survivorship Support:**

- **Transition to Survivorship:** Counseling support goes beyond the treatment period into survivorship, helping patients adjust to life following breast cancer therapy. Counselors support patients in confronting worries of recurrence, managing survivorship-related issues, and enjoying life with renewed purpose, resilience, and optimism.

- **Long-Term Emotional Wellness:** Counseling enhances long-term emotional well-being and resilience among breast cancer survivors. Counselors assist survivors process their cancer experience, integrate it into their life story, and nurture a sense of post-traumatic growth, empowerment, and significance.

**5. Accessing Counseling Services:**

- **Hospital and Cancer Center Services:** Many hospitals and cancer institutes offer counseling services as part of their complete cancer care programs. Patients can check with their healthcare team about accessible counseling options and how to book an appointment with a counselor or therapist.

- **Community Mental Health Resources:** Community mental health centers, counseling clinics, and nonprofit groups may offer low-cost or sliding-scale counseling services for breast cancer patients who may not have access to counseling via their healthcare provider.

Professional counseling and assistance give crucial support to breast cancer patients as they negotiate the emotional complexity of their diagnosis and treatment. By providing a caring and empathic presence, counselors encourage patients to cope more effectively, make educated decisions, navigate relationships, and embrace life with resilience and optimism throughout their cancer journey and beyond.

# 8.

## CONCLUSION

### Encouragement and Uplifting Perspective

In the face of a breast cancer diagnosis, the path ahead may seem intimidating and riddled with uncertainty. However, among the hardships, there is an abundance of hope, courage, and resilience to be discovered. As we end our investigation of breast cancer and its consequences, it's crucial to underline the significance of encouraging and having an optimistic viewpoint.

Breast cancer is not simply a tale of struggle; it's a narrative of victory, tenacity, and the strength of the human spirit. Throughout our conversation, we've met innumerable tales of strength, tenacity, and camaraderie among breast cancer patients, survivors, caregivers, and healthcare professionals. These tales serve as beacons of hope, motivating us to persist, overcome barriers, and embrace life with newfound vibrancy and purpose.

Encouragement may come in many forms: an encouraging remark from a loved one, a caring gesture from a healthcare practitioner, or a shared moment of understanding with a fellow survivor. It's the combined power of our support networks, the unshakable will to tackle adversity head-on, and the tenacity to rise above adversities that move us ahead on our cancer journey.

Maintaining an upbeat attitude doesn't imply dismissing the hardships or underestimating the effect of breast cancer. Instead, it's about admitting the hardships while choosing to concentrate on the potential, the moments of pleasure, and the accomplishments along the journey. It's about discovering beauty in the middle of turmoil, optimism in the face of despair, and thankfulness for each day that we're given.

As we go on, let us continue to elevate and support one another, celebrate the triumphs, no matter how tiny, and to cling hope even in the darkest of times. Together, with bravery, compassion, and resilience, we can conquer the obstacles of breast cancer and emerge stronger, more resilient, and more appreciative of the great gift of life.

In the journey of breast cancer, let us always remember: where there is hope, there is strength; where there is bravery, there is resilience; and where there is love, there is healing. With support and an optimistic viewpoint, we can confront the difficulties of breast cancer with grace, dignity, and steadfast commitment.